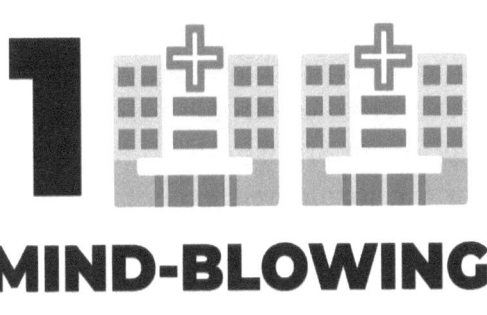

MIND-BLOWING
MEDICAL
BREAKTHROUGHS

100 Life-Changing Discoveries That Saved Millions

FELIX GRAYSON

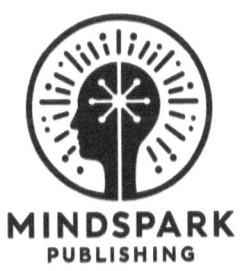

MINDSPARK
PUBLISHING

Published by MindSpark Publishing.
Cover design by MindSpark Publishing.

CONTENTS

BEFORE WE DIVE IN...

Did you know that this is just **one** of many **mind-blowing** books waiting to be discovered?

What if I told you there's a **world of jaw-dropping, unbelievable, and downright bizarre facts** across **sports, science, history, mysteries, and more**—each one packed with stories that will **challenge what you thought you knew?**

EVER WONDERED WHAT IT'S LIKE TO...

- Witness **record-breaking Olympic moments** that defy human limits?

- Explore **real-life conspiracy theories** that sound too wild to be true?

- Discover **unsolved mysteries** that still leave experts baffled?

- Learn about **billionaires, stock market**

crashes, and money secrets?

- Find out how **robots, AI, and space travel are shaping the future?**

- Experience the **most extreme sports, legendary battles, and shocking events?**

This is just the beginning. The **100 Mind-Blowing series** covers it **all.**

WANT TO SEE WHAT'S NEXT?

Go to **FelixGrayson.com** and explore the **growing collection** of books and audiobooks that will **entertain, amaze, and keep you coming back for more.**

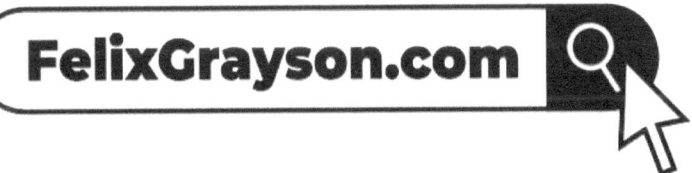

Curiosity doesn't stop here—this is just the beginning. What will blow your mind next?

INTRODUCTION

Welcome to *100 Mind-Blowing Medical Breakthroughs*, a collection designed to make you say, "Wait, that's real science?" From life-saving discoveries to unbelievable innovations, this book is packed with stories that will make you look at medicine in a whole new way.

Have you ever heard of a pill that injects itself? Or a tattoo that monitors your blood sugar? How about a baby cured of HIV, a smart toilet that runs lab tests, or a headset that helps burn victims feel less pain? These are just a few of the jaw-dropping breakthroughs waiting for you inside. Each one has been carefully chosen to surprise, inspire, and maybe even spark a whole new appreciation for how far science has come.

Whether you're here out of curiosity, fascination, or just love sharing wild facts that blow people's minds, this book has something for you. Read it straight through or flip to a random page and see where science takes you.

There's no prescription required—just your curiosity.

So grab a comfy seat, take a deep breath, and get ready to explore some of the most game-changing, life-saving, and downright unbelievable advances in the history of medicine. You just might come away feeling a little more amazed by what the human body—and the human mind—can do. Let's dive in!

Mind-Blowing Medical Breakthrough #1

THE BOY WHO CHANGED POLIO FOREVER

In 1955, the world held its breath as the results of a massive field trial were announced— Jonas Salk's polio vaccine worked. What most people don't know is that the trial involved over **1.8 million children** across the U.S., in what was essentially the largest medical experiment in history. These brave young volunteers were dubbed "Polio Pioneers," and their participation helped prove the vaccine was safe and effective. Within a decade, polio cases in the U.S. dropped by **nearly 90%**, and Salk became an international hero. Even more remarkable? He refused to patent the vaccine, saying it belonged to the people: "Could you patent the sun?"

Mind-Blowing Medical Breakthrough #2

THE ACCIDENTAL CANCER CURE

In the 1940s, doctors studying the effects of **mustard gas** during World War II made a shocking discovery: it **destroyed white blood cells**. This grim finding unexpectedly opened the door to modern chemotherapy. Researchers realized that if a substance could target rapidly dividing cells, it might be used to fight cancers like lymphoma. The result? The first ever **chemotherapy treatments**—born from the wreckage of chemical warfare. What was once a weapon of mass destruction became a life-saving medical breakthrough that has since helped millions battle cancer.

Mind-Blowing Medical Breakthrough #3

THE HEART THAT BEAT OUTSIDE THE BODY

In 1982, a dentist named Barney Clark became the first human to receive a **permanent artificial heart**. The device, called the **Jarvik-7**, was a clunky, humming machine powered by an external air compressor—and yet, it kept Clark alive for **112 days**. Though not a long-term fix, his groundbreaking surgery marked a turning point in medical engineering. For the first time, a human heart could be **replaced** by a man-made machine. Today's versions are far more advanced, but it all started with one bold patient, one plastic heart, and a team willing to defy nature.

Mind-Blowing Medical Breakthrough #4

THE WOMAN WHO MADE CELLS IMMORTAL

In 1951, a woman named **Henrietta Lacks** unknowingly changed medicine forever. Doctors at Johns Hopkins took a small sample of her cancer cells—without her consent—and discovered something astonishing: her cells **didn't die**. Unlike typical cells, Henrietta's continued to divide endlessly, becoming the world's first **immortal cell line**, known as **HeLa cells**. Since then, her cells have been used in **over 75,000 medical studies**, helping to develop vaccines, cancer treatments, gene mapping, and even IVF. Henrietta never knew it, but her cells became one of the most important tools in medical history.

Mind-Blowing Medical Breakthrough #5

THE X-RAY THAT STARTED BY MISTAKE

In 1895, German physicist **Wilhelm Röntgen** was experimenting with cathode rays when he noticed something strange—his screen began to glow **through solid objects**. What he had accidentally discovered was a new kind of invisible light: the **X-ray**. Within weeks, doctors were using it to **see inside the human body** for the first time in history. Röntgen's wife even became the first X-ray subject when he imaged her hand—rings and all. The medical world was forever changed, and Röntgen, refusing to patent the discovery, let the entire world benefit from his unexpected breakthrough.

Mind-Blowing Medical Breakthrough #6

THE BABY SAVED BY BLUE LIGHT

In the 1950s, nurses at a hospital in England noticed something odd: jaundiced newborns placed near **sunny windows** seemed to recover faster. Curious, doctors began testing this and discovered that **blue light** could break down excess bilirubin in the blood—a key cause of jaundice. This accidental observation led to the development of **phototherapy**, a treatment that has since saved **millions of newborns** around the world. Today, the gentle glow of a blue light unit is a standard, life-saving part of neonatal care—all thanks to sunlight and a few observant nurses.

Mind-Blowing Medical Breakthrough #7

THE VACCINE GROWN ON A SLICE OF SKIN

In the 1930s, virologist **Ernest Goodpasture** made a breakthrough using something no one had thought to try: **a fertilized chicken egg**. By injecting viruses into the **membrane lining** just beneath the eggshell, he discovered a way to grow viruses safely outside the human body. This method became the foundation for developing **vaccines** against yellow fever, influenza, and more. In fact, many flu vaccines are **still made this way today**. It all started with a microscope, a cracked egg, and a scientist who dared to look where no one else had.

Mind-Blowing Medical Breakthrough #8

THE MAN WHO SAW HIS OWN BRAIN

In 1971, British engineer **Godfrey Hounsfield** unveiled a machine that could do what no medical device ever had: **create a detailed image of the inside of the human body without cutting it open**. It was the world's first **CT scanner**. To prove it worked, Hounsfield actually scanned his own brain—and the images stunned doctors. Suddenly, they could see tumors, bleeds, and injuries in **three-dimensional detail**. The CT scan revolutionized diagnostics overnight and became one of the most important tools in modern medicine. And yes, the first patient was the inventor himself.

Mind-Blowing Medical Breakthrough #9

THE STOMACH ULCER BACTERIA BOMBSHELL

For decades, doctors believed **stress and spicy food** caused stomach ulcers—until two Australian scientists flipped the script. In the 1980s, **Dr. Barry Marshall** and **Dr. Robin Warren** discovered that most ulcers were actually caused by a bacterium called **Helicobacter pylori**. To prove it, Marshall took the wild step of **drinking a beaker of the bacteria himself**, deliberately infecting his stomach—and developing gastritis. It worked. Their research **revolutionized ulcer treatment**, turning a once-chronic condition into something easily cured with antibiotics. They later won the **Nobel Prize**, but not before one of them became his own test subject.

Mind-Blowing Medical Breakthrough #10

THE BLOOD THAT COULDN'T BE MIXED

In 1901, Austrian doctor **Karl Landsteiner** made a puzzling observation: some blood transfusions saved lives, while others caused deadly reactions. He discovered that human blood comes in different **types**, and mixing the wrong ones can be fatal. His work led to the identification of the **ABO blood group system**, making safe transfusions possible for the first time. Before this, blood transfusion was basically a gamble. Landsteiner's breakthrough laid the foundation for **modern transfusion medicine**, and he later won a **Nobel Prize** for figuring out why blood compatibility matters so much.

Mind-Blowing Medical Breakthrough #11

THE SLEEPING SICKNESS THAT WASN'T

In the early 1960s, doctors in Japan noticed something strange: thousands of women were giving birth to babies with **severe birth defects**, but no one knew why. After intense investigation, the culprit was found—**thalidomide**, a drug marketed to treat morning sickness. Though initially praised as a wonder drug, thalidomide caused **limb deformities and organ damage** in thousands of newborns across the world. The disaster sparked a global reckoning in pharmaceutical safety and led to the creation of **stricter drug approval laws**, especially in the U.S. It was a tragedy—but it also reshaped how we protect patients forever.

Mind-Blowing Medical Breakthrough #12

THE ORGAN THAT GREW IN A LAB

In 1999, scientists at Wake Forest University achieved something once thought to belong in science fiction: they **grew a human bladder in a lab**. Using a patient's own cells and a specially designed scaffold, they were able to construct a working organ and **implant it successfully**. This marked one of the first true successes in **regenerative medicine**. Since then, researchers have created lab-grown windpipes, blood vessels, and even heart tissue—all sparked by that first bioengineered bladder. The dream of growing replacement parts is no longer a dream. It's science—and it's already saving lives.

Mind-Blowing Medical Breakthrough #13

THE COCHLEAR SPARK OF SOUND

In 1978, a man who had been completely deaf for years heard **a beeping noise**—thanks to a revolutionary device implanted in his ear. It was the **first successful cochlear implant**, and it didn't just amplify sound like a hearing aid—it **bypassed damaged parts of the ear** and directly stimulated the auditory nerve. Over time, the technology improved to the point where **speech and music** became recognizable. What began as a series of electronic blips became a **lifeline to sound** for hundreds of thousands of people. The implant redefined what was possible for those living in silence.

Mind-Blowing Medical Breakthrough #14

THE GLUE THAT SEALS WITHOUT STITCHES

Inspired by how **slugs** stick to wet surfaces, scientists in the 2010s developed a **surgical glue** that can seal wounds—even on **beating hearts**. Traditional stitches and staples don't always work well on slippery or moving tissues, but this bio-inspired adhesive forms a tight seal in seconds, flexes with the body, and naturally dissolves over time. Known as **MeTro glue**, it could revolutionize emergency surgery and trauma care, especially in war zones or remote areas. What started with a slimy slug became a breakthrough that's literally holding lives together.

Mind-Blowing Medical Breakthrough #15

THE RETINA PRINTED LIKE INK

In 2018, researchers at the University of Minnesota used a **custom-built 3D printer** to print a sheet of **light-sensitive cells** onto a curved surface—essentially creating a **bionic eye prototype**. While it wasn't yet functional vision, it was the first step toward **printing human retinas**, offering hope to millions affected by blindness. The breakthrough opened the door to future implants that could **restore sight**, and it proved that bioprinting complex, curved tissues wasn't just possible—it was happening. What used to be sci-fi is now staring back with real potential.

Mind-Blowing Medical Breakthrough #16

THE ROBOT THAT PERFORMS SURGERY

In 2000, the FDA approved the **da Vinci Surgical System**, a robot-assisted platform that could perform incredibly precise procedures through tiny incisions. Controlled by a surgeon at a console, da Vinci translated hand movements into **microscopic actions**, reducing blood loss, pain, and recovery time. What once required large open surgeries could now be done with **robotic arms** and a few small cuts. Today, robotic surgery is used for everything from prostate removals to heart valve repairs — making one of the biggest surgical revolutions of the century look like something straight out of Star Wars.

Mind-Blowing Medical Breakthrough #17

THE GENE THAT SWITCHED OFF DISEASE

In 2006, scientists achieved a stunning mile-stone: they used **RNA interference (RNAi)** to **silence a specific gene** in humans for the first time. This meant they could effectively "turn off" the production of disease-causing proteins at the genetic level—without altering the DNA itself. RNAi had been discovered in the late '90s, but this breakthrough showed it could work in real patients. It laid the groundwork for new treatments for **rare genetic disorders**, cancers, and even viral infections. For the first time, medicine could **mute** a gene like hitting pause on a remote control.

Mind-Blowing Medical Breakthrough #18

THE BONE THAT GREW FROM POWDER

In the early 2000s, scientists developed a **synthetic bone graft material** that could be molded like clay and then **harden inside the body**—turning into real bone over time. Made from calcium phosphate, the same mineral found in human bones, this "bone putty" could fill gaps from injuries or surgeries and be gradually replaced by the patient's own living tissue. Unlike traditional metal implants or harvested bone, this **bioactive material** promotes natural healing and reduces rejection. It's not just a filler—it's a scaffold for regeneration. Bone, grown from powder, rebuilding itself from the inside out.

Mind-Blowing Medical Breakthrough #19

THE PILL THAT WATCHES YOU SWALLOW

In 2017, the FDA approved the first **digital pill**—a medication with a tiny **ingestible sensor** that activates when it reaches the stomach. Once swallowed, the pill sends a signal to a wearable patch and smartphone app, confirming the medication was taken. It was initially approved for certain psychiatric conditions where **medication adherence** is critical. While controversial for privacy reasons, the technology opened the door to **smart pharmaceuticals** that could track dosage, monitor response, and improve outcomes. The future of medicine isn't just in the pill—it's what the pill knows.

Mind-Blowing Medical Breakthrough #20

THE CANCER SCANNER IN A DROP OF BLOOD

In 2018, researchers made headlines with a test that could detect **multiple types of cancer** from just a **single drop of blood**. Known as a **liquid biopsy**, this technique identifies fragments of tumor DNA circulating in the bloodstream—often before symptoms even appear. Unlike traditional biopsies, which require surgery or invasive procedures, liquid biopsies are **quick, painless, and repeatable**. They've already begun transforming cancer detection, monitoring, and treatment plans. One drop. That's all it takes to spot a silent killer early—and possibly save a life.

Mind-Blowing Medical Breakthrough #21

THE ARM THAT FELT TOUCH AGAIN

In 2014, scientists unveiled a **mind-controlled prosthetic arm** that didn't just move—it could **feel**. Using electrodes connected directly to the nervous system, the prosthetic sent signals back to the brain, allowing the wearer to **sense pressure and texture** in real time. This was the first time a robotic limb had provided anything close to natural touch, restoring not just motion but sensation. For amputees, it meant regaining something deeply human. A handshake, the feel of a loved one's hand—suddenly possible again, thanks to an arm wired for both strength and feeling.

Mind-Blowing Medical Breakthrough #22

THE SKIN THAT HEALED LIKE WOLVERINE

In 2017, researchers in Japan and the U.S. developed a **spray-on skin** made from stem cells that could **regenerate damaged tissue** in severe burn victims. When sprayed onto a wound, the solution quickly formed a layer of new skin, dramatically speeding up healing and reducing the need for painful grafts. In some cases, patients saw significant recovery in just days. Inspired by comic book superheroes, this breakthrough in **tissue engineering** brought science one step closer to real-life regenerative healing. No claws required—just a spray can and a stem cell solution.

Mind-Blowing Medical Breakthrough #23

THE PARALYZED MAN WHO TOOK A STEP

In 2018, a man paralyzed from the waist down made headlines by **taking steps again**—thanks to a breakthrough in **spinal cord stimulation**. Doctors implanted electrodes near his damaged spinal cord and used targeted electrical pulses to **reawaken dormant neural pathways**. With intense physical therapy and the device's help, he regained partial control over his legs. This wasn't science fiction—it was the beginning of a new era in treating paralysis. From complete immobility to **voluntary movement**, his steps proved the spinal cord can sometimes remember how to walk—with the right kind of nudge.

Mind-Blowing Medical Breakthrough #24

THE LAB TEST ON A PAPER STRIP

In the early 2000s, researchers developed a **paper-based diagnostic test** that could detect diseases like HIV, malaria, and Ebola using just a **drop of blood or saliva**. Inspired by the simplicity of pregnancy tests, these **color-changing strips** required no electricity, refrigeration, or lab equipment—making them perfect for use in **remote or low-resource areas**. Fast, cheap, and incredibly easy to use, these tests revolutionized global health screening and outbreak response. Sometimes, all it takes to save a life is a strip of paper and a splash of science.

Mind-Blowing Medical Breakthrough #25

THE EAR GROWN ON A MOUSE'S BACK

In 1997, a photo stunned the world: a **human-shaped ear** growing on the **back of a lab mouse**. It wasn't fake—it was science. Researchers at Massachusetts General Hospital had used a biodegradable scaffold, seeded with living cartilage cells, to shape the ear. The mouse's body provided the blood supply needed for it to grow. Though the mouse didn't hear a thing, this bizarre and brilliant experiment proved that **human body parts could be grown biologically**. It was a weird sight—but a massive leap for **tissue engineering and reconstructive surgery**.

Mind-Blowing Medical Breakthrough #26

THE DIABETES MONITOR WITHOUT NEEDLES

In 2017, the FDA approved the first **continuous glucose monitor (CGM)** that required **no finger pricks**—a game-changer for people with diabetes. The small sensor, worn on the skin, measured glucose levels in real time and sent updates to a smartphone or reader. No more routine needle sticks, no more guesswork—just a steady stream of life-saving data. The tech gave patients **freedom, control, and peace of mind**, and paved the way for fully automated insulin delivery systems. For millions, it turned managing diabetes from a daily struggle into something far more livable.

Mind-Blowing Medical Breakthrough #27

THE NOSE THAT SMELLED DISEASE

Dogs have been sniffing out disease for years, but in 2020, scientists developed an **electronic nose**—a device that can detect diseases like **lung cancer and Parkinson's** just by analyzing a person's breath. These high-tech sensors pick up on unique chemical patterns, called **volatile organic compounds (VOCs)**, released by the body during illness. With accuracy rates nearing traditional lab tests, this noninvasive tool could one day **replace biopsies and blood draws** for early screening. Imagine walking into a clinic, breathing into a machine—and catching a deadly disease before it even starts.

Mind-Blowing Medical Breakthrough #28

THE PRINTER THAT MADE HUMAN SKIN

In 2019, scientists unveiled a **handheld 3D bioprinter** that could print **layers of human skin directly onto wounds**. Designed for burn victims and deep injuries, the device used a patient's own cells to create custom patches of skin **on the spot**—no need for painful grafts. Unlike traditional printing, this bioprinter adjusted in real time to the wound's shape and depth, making it incredibly precise. Within minutes, it could lay down living tissue that began healing almost immediately. A printer in your hand. Real skin on demand. The future of wound care—layer by layer.

Mind-Blowing Medical Breakthrough #29

THE PACEMAKER POWERED BY HEARTBEATS

In 2021, researchers developed a tiny **energy-harvesting device** that could power a pacemaker using the heart's own **rhythmic motion**. Traditional pacemakers rely on batteries that need surgical replacement every 5–15 years, but this new tech converted the mechanical energy of each heartbeat into **electrical energy**—no batteries required. Still in early stages, the innovation promises a future where **self-charging implants** reduce surgeries and extend device lifespans dramatically. Your heart keeps you alive—and now, it could keep its own support system running too.

Mind-Blowing
Medical Breakthrough
#30

THE CRISPR BABY BREAKTHROUGH

In 2018, a Chinese scientist stunned the world by announcing the birth of the **first gene-edited babies**. Using a revolutionary tool called **CRISPR-Cas9**, he altered the embryos' DNA to make them resistant to HIV before they were born. The experiment triggered global debate and intense ethical backlash—but it proved that **human gene editing** wasn't theoretical anymore. CRISPR, originally discovered as part of a bacterial immune system, had suddenly become one of the most powerful tools in medical history. The age of designer medicine—and controversy—had officially begun.

Mind-Blowing Medical Breakthrough #31

THE PILL THAT REPLACED A LIFETIME

In 2013, a revolutionary cure emerged for **hepatitis C**, a virus that had plagued over 70 million people worldwide. Unlike previous treatments, which involved **painful injections and years of therapy**, this new antiviral pill—**sofosbuvir**—could **completely eliminate the virus in just 8–12 weeks**. With cure rates above 95%, it transformed hep C from a chronic, life-threatening disease into something **quickly and quietly curable**. One pill a day. No injections. No long-term suffering. A lifetime of illness, wiped out with a few weeks of science.

Mind-Blowing Medical Breakthrough #32

THE HELMET THAT REWIRES THE BRAIN

In recent years, doctors have begun treating **depression** using a device that looks more like something from a sci-fi film than a hospital: a **magnetic helmet**. This therapy, called **Transcranial Magnetic Stimulation (TMS)**, delivers focused magnetic pulses to specific regions of the brain—essentially **rebooting faulty neural circuits** linked to mood disorders. For patients who don't respond to medication, TMS has offered **real relief** without surgery or drugs. No scalpels, no chemicals—just magnetism reshaping the mind, one pulse at a time.

Mind-Blowing Medical Breakthrough #33

THE AI THAT OUTDIAGNOSED DOCTORS

In 2016, Google's DeepMind developed an AI system that could analyze **eye scans** with astonishing accuracy—matching or even **surpassing human specialists** in detecting over 50 sight-threatening conditions. Trained on thousands of retinal images, the AI could flag subtle signs of disease **in seconds**, offering faster, earlier diagnosis than many traditional methods. This marked a turning point: artificial intelligence wasn't just assisting—it was **diagnosing**. From eye disease to cancer and beyond, machines are now reading scans, spotting patterns, and saving lives with superhuman precision.

Mind-Blowing Medical Breakthrough #34

THE VACCINE MADE IN RECORD TIME

In 2020, scientists achieved what once seemed impossible: they developed, tested, and rolled out a **safe and effective COVID-19 vaccine** in under **one year**. Traditional vaccine development takes a decade or more—but using **mRNA technology**, companies like Pfizer-BioNTech and Moderna created vaccines that could be rapidly designed and mass-produced. This wasn't just a response to a global crisis—it was a **medical moonshot** that saved millions of lives and showcased the power of modern biotech. Fast, precise, and adaptable, mRNA changed how we fight pandemics forever.

Mind-Blowing Medical Breakthrough #35

THE EXOSKELETON THAT HELPED PEOPLE WALK

In the 2010s, engineers developed wearable **robotic exoskeletons** that allowed people with spinal cord injuries to **stand, walk, and climb stairs**—sometimes for the first time in years. These battery-powered suits used sensors, motors, and AI to mimic natural movement, responding to subtle shifts in the user's weight and balance. Originally built for rehabilitation, exoskeletons are now being used in hospitals, homes, and even workplaces. It's not just about mobility—it's about **dignity and independence**, powered by a suit of steel and smarts.

Mind-Blowing Medical Breakthrough #36

THE CONTACT LENS THAT DETECTS DISEASE

In a remarkable fusion of tech and biology, scientists have created **smart contact lenses** that can **monitor health in real time**. These lenses can detect changes in **glucose levels, eye pressure, and even cancer biomarkers**— all through your tears. Some prototypes are equipped with micro-LEDs and wireless transmitters, turning the eye into a live data stream. For people with diabetes or glaucoma, this means continuous, noninvasive monitoring with zero finger pricks or bulky machines. It's not just vision correction anymore—your contacts might soon **diagnose disease before symptoms appear**.

Mind-Blowing Medical Breakthrough #37

THE ORGANS KEPT ALIVE IN A BOX

For decades, donated organs had to be transplanted within hours—kept on ice and racing against the clock. But in the 2010s, doctors introduced **organ perfusion machines**—devices that **keep hearts, lungs, and livers warm, oxygenated, and even beating** outside the body. Dubbed "organs on life support," these machines can **extend viability for transplant up to 24 hours** or more. Some organs have even improved during transport. More time means more lives saved—and it's all thanks to a box that doesn't just preserve organs... it **keeps them alive**.

Mind-Blowing Medical Breakthrough #38

THE MIRROR THAT MONITORS YOUR HEALTH

In recent years, tech innovators have developed **smart mirrors** that do more than reflect your face—they can **track vital signs** like heart rate, respiratory rate, and even emotional stress using subtle changes in skin tone and facial movement. Some versions can integrate with wearables, suggest personalized health tips, and flag early signs of illness—all while you brush your teeth. It's like having a **mini checkup every morning,** no appointments required. The bathroom mirror is no longer just a reflection—it's a silent partner in preventive care.

Mind-Blowing Medical Breakthrough #39

THE APP THAT DIAGNOSED SKIN CANCER

In the 2020s, dermatology took a digital leap with **AI-powered smartphone apps** that could **analyze moles and skin lesions** using just a photo. Trained on millions of images, these apps could identify signs of melanoma and other skin cancers with **remarkable accuracy**, offering instant results and prompting early medical follow-up. For people in remote areas—or those who might otherwise delay care—this meant faster, potentially life-saving detection. The dermatologist in your pocket might not wear a white coat, but it **just might save your life**.

Mind-Blowing Medical Breakthrough #40

THE PILL CAMERA THAT EXPLORES YOUR GUT

In 2001, medicine took a tiny leap forward—literally—with the debut of the **capsule endoscope**: a pill-sized camera that patients **swallow** to capture thousands of images as it travels through the digestive tract. This noninvasive marvel made it possible to explore the **small intestine**, a region once nearly impossible to examine without surgery. No tubes, no sedation—just a smooth ride and a stream of high-res photos. For diagnosing conditions like Crohn's disease or bleeding ulcers, the tiny explorer opened a **huge window into hidden parts of the body**.

Mind-Blowing Medical Breakthrough #41

THE GENE MAP THAT CHANGED EVERYTHING

In 2003, after 13 years of global effort, scientists completed the **Human Genome Project**—a complete map of all **3 billion base pairs** that make up human DNA. For the first time, we had a full blueprint of the human body's genetic code. This breakthrough launched a revolution in **personalized medicine**, allowing doctors to predict disease risk, tailor treatments, and understand the genetic roots of countless conditions. It didn't just answer age-old questions—it opened thousands of new ones. The book of life had been read cover to cover—and we were just getting started.

Mind-Blowing Medical Breakthrough #42

THE BREAST CANCER CHIP THAT SPEEDS RESULTS

In the early 2020s, scientists developed a **microfluidic chip** that could test breast cancer biopsies **faster and more accurately** than traditional lab methods. This tiny device, often smaller than a credit card, used fluid dynamics to isolate and analyze tumor cells in real time—delivering diagnostic insights in **hours instead of days**. Faster results meant quicker treatment decisions, less waiting, and improved outcomes. It's a breakthrough that shrunk the lab down to a chip—and put precious time back into the hands of patients and doctors.

Mind-Blowing Medical Breakthrough #43

THE WATCH THAT CALLS FOR HELP

What started as a fitness tracker quickly became a **life-saving device**. In 2018, smartwatches like the Apple Watch introduced features like **fall detection** and **irregular heartbeat alerts**. If a user took a hard fall and didn't respond within seconds, the watch could automatically **call emergency services** and share their location. For many—especially seniors or heart patients—this meant help could arrive even if they couldn't speak or move. It's not just wearable tech anymore. It's a silent guardian, waiting on your wrist to step in when you can't.

Mind-Blowing
Medical Breakthrough
#44

THE BLOOD TEST THAT PREDICTS ALZHEIMER'S

In 2020, researchers unveiled a simple **blood test** that could detect early signs of **Alzheimer's disease**—years before symptoms appeared. By measuring levels of specific proteins linked to brain degeneration, the test could predict with over **90% accuracy** whether someone was likely to develop the disease. Until then, diagnosis required expensive brain scans or spinal taps. This breakthrough promised a future where **early detection** and **prevention strategies** could start long before memory fades. One vial of blood. A glimpse into the brain's future—and a fighting chance to change it.

Mind-Blowing
Medical Breakthrough
#45

THE TATTOO THAT TRACKS YOUR HEALTH

Scientists have developed **biosensing tattoos**—special inks that **change color in response to changes inside the body**, like glucose levels, dehydration, or electrolyte imbalance. These tattoos aren't just for decoration—they act like **real-time medical monitors**, turning the skin into a live dashboard for health. One version shifts from green to brown as blood sugar rises, offering a noninvasive way to track diabetes. Another glows under UV light to show sodium levels. With just a glance at your arm, you could soon check your health **without a single needle or screen**.

Mind-Blowing Medical Breakthrough #46

THE VOICE THAT DIAGNOSED DISEASE

In recent years, researchers have discovered that **your voice** can reveal far more than mood—it can also signal **diseases like Parkinson's, depression, and even COVID-19**. By analyzing vocal patterns, breathing, tone, and rhythm, AI-powered tools have been trained to detect subtle changes linked to specific conditions. Some apps can flag issues **before physical symptoms appear**, simply by listening to a short voice recording. It's a futuristic stethoscope you don't wear, touch, or see—just **speak**, and your body might tell a story your ears can't hear.

Mind-Blowing Medical Breakthrough #47

THE NOSE SPRAY THAT STOPS PARALYSIS

In a stunning 2021 study, scientists developed a **nasal spray** that helped **paralyzed mice walk again**—within hours. The spray delivered a designer protein that **repaired damaged spinal cord tissue** by promoting cell regeneration and reconnecting severed nerves. While still in experimental stages, the breakthrough hinted at a future where a simple, noninvasive treatment could one day help humans **recover from devastating spinal injuries**. No surgery. No implants. Just a mist up the nose—with the power to reboot the body's broken wiring.

Mind-Blowing Medical Breakthrough #48

THE HOSPITAL THAT FITS IN A BACKPACK

In emergency zones and disaster areas, bulky medical gear can mean the difference between life and death. That's why engineers created an **ultra-portable hospital-in-a-backpack**—a compact kit equipped with **solar-powered devices**, diagnostics, medications, and even a small surgical suite. Designed for use in remote or war-torn regions, it allows frontline medics to deliver **critical care on the move**, without waiting for infrastructure. One backpack. One responder. Dozens of lives saved. It's the ER that goes where ambulances can't.

Mind-Blowing Medical Breakthrough #49

THE TOOTH THAT REGREW ITSELF

In 2023, scientists in Japan announced a clinical trial for a **drug that could regrow human teeth**—no implants or dentures required. The treatment targets a specific protein that suppresses tooth growth, allowing **dormant "tooth buds"** to activate and form entirely new teeth. Originally tested in ferrets and mice, the results were so promising that trials on humans began shortly after. If successful, it could mark the end of artificial dental replacements. Imagine losing a tooth... and **growing a brand new one**, just like sharks do.

Mind-Blowing Medical Breakthrough #50

THE CANCER DRUG THAT VANISHED TUMORS

In 2022, a small clinical trial stunned the medical world: **every single patient's tumor disappeared**. The trial used a targeted immunotherapy drug called **dostarlimab**, which helps the immune system **unmask and destroy cancer cells**. It was tested on patients with a specific type of rectal cancer, and all 18 participants saw **complete remission**—no chemo, no surgery, no radiation. While more research is needed, it marked one of the most dramatic responses ever seen in oncology. A cancer treatment where the body fights back—and **wins completely**.

Mind-Blowing Medical Breakthrough #51

THE BABY CURED OF HIV

In 2013, doctors made headlines when a baby born with **HIV** was given an aggressive course of antiretroviral drugs **just 30 hours after birth**—and by 18 months, the virus was undetectable **without ongoing treatment**. While not a guaranteed cure, the case offered stunning hope that **early intervention** could prevent HIV from taking hold in newborns. It challenged everything doctors thought they knew about the virus's grip on the body—and cracked open the door to a future where **HIV transmission at birth could be stopped in its tracks**.

Mind-Blowing Medical Breakthrough #52

THE FINGER THAT GREW BACK

In the mid-2000s, a man who lost the tip of his finger in a model plane accident was treated with a powdered substance known as **"pixie dust"**—actually made from **pig bladder extracellular matrix**. Applied to the wound, the matrix acted as a biological scaffold, encouraging the body to **regrow skin, tissue, and even nail**. Within weeks, the fingertip had **regenerated completely**. Though still experimental, this regenerative technique hinted at a future where limbs, not just cells, might be **coaxed back to life with the right biological cue**.

Mind-Blowing Medical Breakthrough #53

THE BRAIN IMPLANT THAT TREATS ADDICTION

In 2020, surgeons in China implanted a tiny **deep brain stimulation (DBS) device** into a man battling severe opioid addiction. The device delivered controlled electrical pulses to targeted areas of the brain involved in **craving and reward**. Remarkably, the patient reported a dramatic drop in drug urges—and similar trials soon followed in other countries. While DBS has been used for Parkinson's and depression, its application in addiction opened up **a bold new frontier**. It's not a cure-all, but for some, a few milliamps might mean the difference between relapse and recovery.

Mind-Blowing Medical Breakthrough #54

THE MIRROR THERAPY THAT FOOLED THE BRAIN

In the 1990s, a simple box with mirrors launched a medical breakthrough. Known as **mirror therapy**, it was used to treat patients with **phantom limb pain**—a condition where amputees feel pain in a missing limb. By placing their intact limb in front of a mirror, patients created the illusion that both limbs were present and moving. Amazingly, this visual trick **retrained the brain** and often **reduced or eliminated pain**. No drugs. No surgery. Just the power of perception rewiring the mind to let go of pain that no longer had a source.

Mind-Blowing Medical Breakthrough #55

THE HOSPITAL ROOM THAT HEALS FASTER

In the 2010s, hospitals began redesigning patient rooms with **healing architecture**—using elements like **natural light, noise control, views of nature, and calming colors**. Studies showed that patients in these optimized environments experienced **faster recovery times, lower stress levels, and reduced need for pain medication**. One famous study even found that patients with a window view of trees healed faster than those facing a brick wall. It turns out, medicine isn't always something you swallow—sometimes, it's **the room you're in that makes you better**.

Mind-Blowing Medical Breakthrough #56

THE 3D-PRINTED SPINE IMPLANT

In 2014, a 12-year-old boy in China became the first patient to receive a **3D-printed vertebra**, replacing a damaged section of his spine caused by cancer. Custom-designed from medical scans and printed in titanium, the implant fit **perfectly** into his neck and allowed natural bone to **grow into it over time**. Unlike traditional implants, it required no screws or cement. It was a stunning debut for 3D printing in complex, load-bearing surgeries—and it proved that the future of spinal repair might be built **layer by layer, just for you**.

Mind-Blowing Medical Breakthrough #57

THE EYE DROPS THAT REPLACE READING GLASSES

In 2021, the FDA approved a new kind of eye drop—**Vuity**—that could temporarily **sharpen near vision** for adults with age-related farsightedness (presbyopia). Just one drop in each eye could improve close-up focus for **6 to 10 hours**, reducing or even eliminating the need for reading glasses. The drops work by constricting the pupil, enhancing depth of focus naturally. For millions tired of fumbling for specs at restaurants or reading labels at arm's length, it was a tiny squirt with a huge payoff—**clear vision, no glasses required**.

Mind-Blowing Medical Breakthrough #58

THE BREATHALYZER THAT DETECTS DIABETES

Long before symptoms appear, people with undiagnosed diabetes can exhale a subtle, fruity odor—caused by **acetone** in the breath. In the 2020s, scientists developed a **noninvasive breathalyzer** that can detect this marker with high accuracy, offering a painless alternative to blood tests. The device analyzes the air you exhale and delivers results in minutes, making it ideal for **early screening and real-time monitoring**. One deep breath could soon reveal what's happening in your bloodstream—**no needles, no strips, just science in the air**.

Mind-Blowing Medical Breakthrough #59

THE LAB-GROWN BLOOD FOR TRANSFUSIONS

In a groundbreaking 2022 trial, scientists in the UK successfully **created red blood cells in a lab** and transfused them into humans for the first time. Grown from donated stem cells, this lab-made blood aimed to help patients with **rare blood types** who often struggle to find compatible donors. Unlike donated blood, these manufactured cells can be tailored for perfect matches and may even **last longer in the body**. It's a bold leap toward a future where blood shortages fade—and **transfusions come from petri dishes, not people**.

Mind-Blowing Medical Breakthrough #60

THE ULTRASOUND THAT ZAPS TUMORS

In the 2020s, doctors began using a technique called **focused ultrasound** to treat tumors and other conditions **without surgery or radiation**. By directing high-frequency sound waves to a precise spot in the body, they could **heat and destroy diseased tissue**—all through intact skin. It's already being used to treat **essential tremor, prostate cancer, and uterine fibroids**, with clinical trials expanding fast. No cuts. No recovery rooms. Just sound waves doing surgical work **from the outside in**—quietly, painlessly, and with remarkable precision.

Mind-Blowing Medical Breakthrough #61

THE SMART BANDAGE THAT TALKS BACK

In 2022, researchers introduced a **smart bandage** that not only covers wounds—but **monitors healing and delivers treatment** as needed. Equipped with tiny sensors, the bandage tracks things like **temperature, pH, and oxygen levels**, alerting doctors if an infection is forming. Some versions even release medication or use gentle electrical stimulation to **speed up tissue repair**. It's a bandage that doesn't just sit there—it **thinks, adapts, and heals**. The age of passive wound care is over—your bandage is now part of the medical team.

Mind-Blowing Medical Breakthrough #62

THE AI NURSE THAT NEVER SLEEPS

Hospitals around the world are starting to deploy **virtual AI nurses**, like "Moxi" and "Florence," that assist with **routine tasks**—delivering supplies, answering patient questions, and even monitoring vital signs. These robotic helpers free up human staff for more critical care, reducing burnout and improving efficiency. Some systems even use **natural language processing** to have friendly, comforting conversations with patients—day or night. They don't replace doctors, but they do lighten the load. Always on call, never tired—**the nurse that works 24/7 without blinking**.

Mind-Blowing Medical Breakthrough #63

THE NEEDLE THAT FINDS THE VEIN ITSELF

For patients who fear needles—or have hard-to-find veins—a new device is changing the game. Using **near-infrared light and AI**, this smart injection system can **map veins in real time** and guide the needle with incredible accuracy, drastically reducing failed attempts. Some systems even use robotic arms to insert the needle automatically. Originally developed for pediatric and cancer patients, it's now spreading across hospitals and labs. No more multiple jabs or guesswork—just **a needle that knows exactly where to go**.

Mind-Blowing Medical Breakthrough #64

THE SURGERY GUIDED BY AUGMENTED REALITY

In a futuristic fusion of tech and medicine, surgeons are now using **augmented reality (AR) headsets** to overlay **3D images of organs, bones, and tumors** directly onto the patient's body during surgery. These AR systems, like Microsoft's HoloLens, provide real-time guidance, allowing doctors to "see" beneath the skin without making a cut. It boosts precision, shortens procedures, and reduces complications. What once lived on scans or monitors now appears right in the surgeon's field of view—**turning anatomy into a live, interactive map.**

Mind-Blowing Medical Breakthrough #65

THE IMPLANT THAT REVERSES BLINDNESS

In a stunning breakthrough, researchers developed a **bionic eye implant** that can partially restore vision in people with severe blindness. The device, called **Argus II**, uses a **tiny camera mounted on glasses** to capture images, which are then converted into electrical signals and sent to an **implant in the retina**. Patients can't see like before—but they can detect light, shapes, and movement, helping them **navigate independently**. It's not a miracle cure, but it's a real, working interface between technology and the brain—**a first glimpse back into the world of sight**.

Mind-Blowing Medical Breakthrough #66

THE PILL THAT MELTS IN YOUR CHEEK

For patients who struggle to swallow pills—especially children, the elderly, or those with neurological conditions—scientists created **orally disintegrating tablets (ODTs)** that **melt instantly** when placed inside the cheek or under the tongue. These fast-acting pills don't require water and begin absorbing **directly into the bloodstream**, offering quicker relief and better compliance. Used for everything from **pain and allergies to seizures and nausea**, they've turned a simple tweak in delivery into a **life-changing innovation in accessibility and speed**. Just place, wait, and heal.

Mind-Blowing Medical Breakthrough #67

THE TOOTHBRUSH THAT DETECTS DISEASE

In the 2020s, engineers unveiled a **smart toothbrush** equipped with **biosensors** that could detect early signs of **gum disease, cavities, and even systemic illnesses** like diabetes—all from saliva analysis during your morning routine. Some models sync with smartphone apps to track brushing habits, flag warning signs, and even remind users to schedule dentist visits. It's preventative care built right into something you already use every day. Brush your teeth, **scan your health**—all in under two minutes.

Mind-Blowing Medical Breakthrough #68

THE JACKET THAT CALMS THE HEART

Originally designed for children with autism, **deep pressure vests**—wearable jackets that apply gentle, constant pressure—have shown surprising benefits for **anxiety, PTSD, and even high blood pressure**. The pressure stimulates the **parasympathetic nervous system**, triggering a calming response similar to a hug. Now adapted for adults and used in hospitals, airports, and therapy sessions, these high-tech garments are helping people manage panic attacks and emotional overload **without medication**. It's like wearing a hug—a simple squeeze with powerful results.

Mind-Blowing Medical Breakthrough #69

THE ROBOT THAT DELIVERS YOUR MEDICATION

Hospitals are now using **autonomous delivery robots** to transport medications, lab samples, and supplies across sprawling medical campuses. These robots—like **TUG** and **Moxi**—navigate hallways, open doors, and even ride elevators on their own, freeing up staff to focus on patient care. Equipped with **secure compartments and sensors**, they ensure critical items arrive safely and on time. They don't get tired, lost, or distracted—just reliable, rolling helpers making healthcare **faster, safer, and smarter**.

Mind-Blowing Medical Breakthrough #70

THE BRAIN SCAN THAT READS THOUGHTS

In a groundbreaking 2023 study, researchers used **fMRI brain scans combined with AI** to **decode complete sentences** from a person's thoughts—without them speaking a word. By analyzing blood flow patterns in specific brain regions, the system could translate neural activity into readable text with surprising accuracy. Though still in early stages, this tech could one day help **paralyzed or nonverbal patients** communicate in real time, simply by thinking. It's not mind reading like in sci-fi—but it's closer than anyone thought possible.

Mind-Blowing Medical Breakthrough #71

THE PHONE THAT DOES AN EYE EXAM

In recent years, scientists developed smart-phone attachments and apps that can perform **comprehensive eye exams**, including tests for **visual acuity, retinal imaging, and even cataracts**. These low-cost tools bring diagnostics to **rural and underserved areas**, where access to ophthalmologists is limited. In minutes, a phone can capture high-resolution images of the eye and send them to specialists for review. What used to require bulky equipment and clinic visits now fits in your pocket—**vision care, delivered through a lens and a swipe.**

Mind-Blowing Medical Breakthrough #72

THE LIGHT THAT HEALS BROKEN BONES

Researchers have discovered that **low-level laser therapy (LLLT)** can **accelerate bone healing** by stimulating cellular activity and increasing blood flow at the injury site. Often referred to as "cold laser" treatment, this painless, noninvasive technique has shown promise in speeding up recovery from **fractures, dental implants, and joint injuries**. It's already being used in sports medicine and orthopedics—with zero drugs, no side effects, and no surgery. Just focused light, turning fractures into fast healers—**like a flashlight aimed at regeneration.**

Mind-Blowing Medical Breakthrough #73

THE SALIVA TEST THAT SPOTS CONCUSSIONS

In the early 2020s, scientists developed a **saliva-based test** that could detect **biomarkers linked to concussions**—within minutes. Originally designed for athletes, the test identifies tiny fragments of **brain-specific RNA** released after head trauma. Unlike traditional concussion assessments, which rely on symptoms and guesswork, this test offers **objective, biological proof** of injury. Quick, portable, and noninvasive, it's transforming how we diagnose and manage brain injuries—**with just a spit sample and a few minutes of science.**

Mind-Blowing Medical Breakthrough #74

THE EXHALED BREATH THAT DETECTS CANCER

In a major leap forward, scientists have created **breathalyzers** that can detect early signs of **lung, stomach, and even ovarian cancer**—just by analyzing the **chemical compounds in exhaled air**. These volatile organic compounds (VOCs) serve as unique "cancer fingerprints," and advanced sensors paired with AI can spot them long before traditional symptoms appear. Noninvasive, fast, and painless, breath diagnostics could soon become routine screenings—**one deep breath, one early warning, one life potentially saved.**

Mind-Blowing Medical Breakthrough #75

THE SMART INHALER THAT TRACKS EVERY BREATH

Asthma and COPD patients often forget or mistime their inhaler doses—but **smart inhalers** are changing that. Equipped with tiny sensors and Bluetooth, these devices **track usage, monitor technique**, and send data to a smartphone app or doctor in real time. Some even use reminders, weather alerts, and personalized tips to prevent attacks before they start. Studies show they dramatically improve medication adherence and reduce hospital visits. It's a breath of fresh air for chronic lung care—**inhalers that treat and teach at the same time.**

Mind-Blowing Medical Breakthrough #76

THE BANDAGE THAT STOPS BLEEDING FAST

Inspired by nature, researchers developed a **gel-infused bandage** that can **stop severe bleeding in under 30 seconds**. Using materials derived from **shrimp shells and algae**, the bandage quickly forms a **sticky, clot-promoting seal** when pressed onto a wound—even in cases of major trauma. Originally designed for battlefield and emergency use, it's now saving lives in ambulances and operating rooms worldwide. It doesn't just cover wounds—it **shuts them down fast**, buying precious time when seconds matter most.

Mind-Blowing Medical Breakthrough #77

THE TOILET THAT ANALYZES YOUR HEALTH

Engineers have developed **smart toilets** that can analyze **urine and stool in real time**, checking for signs of infection, dehydration, kidney disease, and even certain cancers. Some models use embedded sensors, cameras, and AI to track health trends over time—**no effort required** from the user. The goal? Early detection of chronic and life-threatening conditions through a device you use every day. It's the most passive health check imaginable—**your toilet quietly doing diagnostics while you flush.**

Mind-Blowing Medical Breakthrough #78

THE SOUND WAVES THAT HEAL WOUNDS

In a surprising medical twist, scientists discovered that **low-frequency sound waves** can dramatically **accelerate wound healing**. When applied to chronic ulcers or diabetic foot sores, these gentle vibrations stimulate **cell growth, blood flow, and tissue repair**—all without touching the wound. The therapy is painless, noninvasive, and can even help wounds that haven't healed in years. No needles, no scalpels—just a hum of sound coaxing the body to **repair itself faster than ever thought possible.**

Mind-Blowing Medical Breakthrough #79

THE VR HEADSET THAT REDUCES PAIN

Virtual reality isn't just for gaming—it's now used in hospitals to **relieve pain and anxiety**. Studies show that when patients wear a VR headset during procedures like wound care or childbirth, their brains become so **immersed in calming virtual environments** that they experience **less pain and stress**. Some hospitals use it for burn victims, while others use it for phobias, physical therapy, or even chemotherapy sessions. It's a digital escape with real-world results—**a headset that doesn't just distract, it heals.**

Mind-Blowing Medical Breakthrough #80

THE GENE THERAPY THAT FIXED BUBBLE BOY

In 2019, doctors used **gene therapy** to cure infants born with **severe combined immunodeficiency (SCID)**—a rare condition often called "bubble boy disease." By inserting a corrected version of the faulty gene into the child's own stem cells and reinfusing them, doctors were able to **rebuild a functioning immune system** from the inside out. For the first time, these children could leave isolation and face the world safely. It wasn't just a treatment—it was a **genetic reset button** that turned a death sentence into a cure.

Mind-Blowing Medical Breakthrough #81

THE ALGORITHM THAT SPOTS SEPSIS EARLY

Sepsis is one of the leading causes of death in hospitals—but it's notoriously hard to catch in time. In response, researchers developed an **AI-powered early warning system** that monitors patient data in real time—**vitals, lab results, and medical history**—to flag subtle patterns of sepsis hours before symptoms become obvious. Tested in clinical settings, it has already saved lives by **alerting doctors sooner than any human could**. It's a quiet, tireless algorithm working behind the scenes—**finding danger before it becomes deadly.**

Mind-Blowing Medical Breakthrough #82

THE DRONE THAT DELIVERS LIFESAVING BLOOD

In Rwanda and Ghana, drones are now being used to **deliver blood, vaccines, and emergency medicine** to remote areas in a fraction of the time it takes by road. These autonomous aircraft, developed by companies like Zipline, can travel **up to 80 miles round trip**, dropping supplies by parachute within minutes of a request. In some regions, they've **cut delivery times from hours to minutes**—literally saving lives in postpartum hemorrhages and trauma cases. It's high-tech logistics with high-stakes results—**medicine that flies faster than traffic ever could.**

Mind-Blowing Medical Breakthrough #83

THE PILL THAT TREATS POSTPARTUM BLEEDING

Postpartum hemorrhage is one of the **leading causes of maternal death** worldwide—especially in low-resource settings. In response, scientists developed a low-cost, heat-stable pill called **tranexamic acid (TXA)** that can **dramatically reduce bleeding** when given soon after childbirth. Unlike many medications, TXA doesn't need refrigeration and can be **safely used without specialized equipment**, making it ideal for rural clinics and field use. One small tablet, given at the right moment, has the power to **turn childbirth from a crisis into a celebration.**

Mind-Blowing Medical Breakthrough #84

THE SCANNER THAT DIAGNOSES MALARIA FAST

Diagnosing malaria in rural areas used to require microscopes, lab techs, and time. But now, scientists have developed **portable malaria scanners** that use **infrared light or magnetism** to detect infected blood cells in **seconds**—no needles, no reagents, and no expert needed. Some devices work with a simple finger clip, while others scan a drop of blood on a slide. Fast, accurate, and battery-powered, these tools are revolutionizing frontline care in malaria-endemic regions—**bringing high-tech detection to the lowest-resource settings.**

Mind-Blowing Medical Breakthrough #85

THE GLOVE THAT RESTORES HAND MOVEMENT

For stroke survivors and people with neurological injuries, losing hand function can feel permanent. But in the 2020s, engineers created **robotic rehabilitation gloves** that help retrain the brain and muscles through **repetitive, assisted motion**. Worn like a flexible exoskeleton, the glove gently guides fingers through gripping and stretching exercises—sometimes even **responding to brain signals** in real time. With regular use, patients have regained strength, dexterity, and independence. It's not just therapy—it's **hope you can slip on, one finger at a time.**

Mind-Blowing Medical Breakthrough #86

THE T-CELLS TRAINED TO KILL CANCER

In a revolutionary leap for cancer treatment, scientists developed **CAR-T therapy**, which involves extracting a patient's own **T-cells**, genetically modifying them to recognize and attack cancer cells, and then infusing them back into the body. The results have been staggering—**complete remission** in some patients with leukemia and lymphoma who had exhausted all other options. It's like giving your immune system **a custom set of blueprints** to find and destroy the enemy. Not chemotherapy. Not radiation. Just your own cells, **retrained to win the war inside.**

Mind-Blowing Medical Breakthrough #87

THE PACIFIER THAT MONITORS VITAL SIGNS

For premature and newborn babies in the NICU, even the simplest vitals can require bulky, wired monitors. But in 2023, researchers introduced a **smart pacifier** that tracks **heart rate, oxygen levels, and temperature**—all without invasive leads or uncomfortable adhesives. It looks and feels like a regular pacifier, but inside are soft sensors that transmit data wirelessly, giving clinicians a real-time window into infant health. Gentle, noninvasive, and stress-free, it's a comforting innovation where it matters most—**in the smallest patients.**

Mind-Blowing Medical Breakthrough #88

THE PILL THAT TRACKS YOUR GUT JOURNEY

In recent years, researchers developed an **ingestible sensor capsule** that travels through the digestive system, collecting real-time data on **pH, temperature, gas levels, and pressure**. This "smart pill" helps diagnose conditions like **IBS, Crohn's, and motility disorders**—without invasive scopes or imaging. It wirelessly transmits information as it moves, offering a detailed map of your gut's activity from the inside out. One swallow, zero discomfort, and a **complete internal tour on the way out.**

Mind-Blowing Medical Breakthrough #89

THE CHAIR THAT DETECTS HEART TROUBLE

At first glance, it looks like a regular armchair—but built into the cushions are sensors that can **monitor heart rate, blood pressure, and even detect atrial fibrillation**. Designed for elderly or high-risk patients, this **smart chair** passively collects vital signs while the person simply sits and relaxes. No wires, no patches—just data gathered quietly during everyday rest. It's preventive care without interruption, offering doctors a **real-time window into heart health, one sit at a time.**

Mind-Blowing Medical Breakthrough #90

THE APP THAT DETECTS EAR INFECTIONS

In 2019, researchers developed a smartphone app that could **diagnose ear infections** using just a **paper cone and the phone's microphone**. The app plays a soft sound into the ear and analyzes the reflected audio to detect fluid behind the eardrum—a key sign of infection. With accuracy comparable to trained doctors, this tool empowers parents and rural clinics to **catch infections early** without specialized equipment. No scopes, no guesswork—**just a phone, a paper cone, and the science of sound.**

Mind-Blowing Medical Breakthrough #91

THE EYE IMPLANT THAT DRIPS MEDICINE

For patients with chronic eye diseases like **glaucoma or macular degeneration**, daily eye drops can be a hassle—and often missed. Enter the **medication-dispensing eye implant**, a tiny reservoir inserted just under the surface of the eye that **slowly releases drugs over months**. No need to remember doses, and no more fluctuating pressure or symptoms. Just steady, targeted treatment **from the inside out**, giving patients both freedom and better results—**an eye drop you never have to apply.**

Mind-Blowing Medical Breakthrough #92

THE BRACELET THAT PREDICTS ILLNESS

In recent years, wearable devices like **smart health bracelets** have advanced beyond step counting—they can now detect **subtle changes in skin temperature, heart rate variability, and respiration** that may signal infection **days before symptoms appear**. Some studies even showed these wearables could flag COVID-19 or flu **before a person felt sick**, offering a head start on isolation or treatment. It's your body's early-warning system, picked up by a wristband that **notices what you don't—even before you sneeze**.

Mind-Blowing Medical Breakthrough #93

THE WATCH THAT WARNS OF A STROKE

A cutting-edge smartwatch feature now monitors for **atrial fibrillation (AFib)**—a common but often silent heart rhythm disorder that dramatically increases the risk of stroke. When the watch detects irregular rhythms, it alerts the wearer and can even generate an **ECG reading** on the spot, ready to share with a doctor. For many, it's caught the condition early—**before any symptoms ever appeared.** It's not just a gadget anymore—it's a lifesaver that wraps around your wrist and listens for the subtle signs of a future emergency.

Mind-Blowing Medical Breakthrough #94

THE IMPLANT THAT CONTROLS EPILEPSY

For patients with severe epilepsy, doctors have developed a **neurostimulator implant**—often called a **"brain pacemaker"**—that detects the early signs of a seizure and delivers a burst of electrical pulses to **stop it before it starts**. Implanted in the skull and connected to brain tissue, the device learns each patient's unique seizure patterns and adjusts over time. It's already helped thousands reduce seizure frequency and severity. Not a cure, but a **lifeline of electricity**—quietly guarding the brain from within.

Mind-Blowing Medical Breakthrough #95

THE PILL THAT DELIVERS ITSELF WITH A POP

Inspired by the self-righting shape of a leopard tortoise, engineers created a **self-injecting pill** that delivers drugs—like **insulin**—directly into the stomach lining. Once swallowed, the capsule orients itself, uses a tiny spring-loaded microneedle to inject the medication, and then **harmlessly dissolves**. Completely painless and proven safe in early trials, this breakthrough could one day replace daily injections for millions of patients. No more syringes—just a pop, a poke, and **a dose delivered from the inside out.**

Mind-Blowing Medical Breakthrough #96

THE TATTOO THAT MONITORS BLOOD SUGAR

For people with diabetes, finger pricks could soon be a thing of the past. Researchers have developed a **graphene-based tattoo sensor** that sits on the skin and continuously **monitors glucose levels through sweat**, not blood. It's ultra-thin, flexible, and completely painless—transmitting real-time data to a smartphone. Some versions even come with tiny heaters to **stimulate sweat on demand**, ensuring reliable readings. It's discreet, noninvasive, and futuristic—**a health monitor that sticks like ink and thinks like a lab.**

Mind-Blowing Medical Breakthrough #97

THE E-PATCH THAT REPLACES INJECTIONS

Scientists have created **microneedle patch-es**—small, pain-free adhesive strips that deliver medications like vaccines or insulin through **hundreds of microscopic needles** that barely penetrate the skin. They dissolve harmlessly after application and don't require refrigeration, making them perfect for use in **remote or low-resource areas**. Just peel, stick, and wait a few minutes—**no syringes, no fear, no special training required**. It's the future of medicine, packaged like a Band-Aid and worn like progress.

Mind-Blowing Medical Breakthrough #98

THE AI THAT LISTENS FOR CARDIAC ARREST

Researchers have trained smart devices—like smart speakers and phones—to **listen for the distinct gasping sound of agonal breathing**, which often occurs during **cardiac arrest**. When detected, the system can **automatically call emergency services** and provide the exact location, even if the person can't speak or move. Tested in real-world settings, the technology has already proven its potential to **spot medical emergencies faster than people nearby**. It's a life-saving eavesdropper—**always listening, just in case.**

Mind-Blowing Medical Breakthrough #99

THE PILL THAT RECORDS YOUR GUT SOUNDS

Scientists have developed a swallowable capsule that doesn't just travel through the digestive tract—it **records internal sounds**. Equipped with a tiny microphone, the "**acoustic pill**" listens to **gut gurgles, contractions, and motility patterns**, helping doctors diagnose conditions like **IBS, blockages, or gastroparesis**. It's painless, wireless, and offers insights that scopes and scans can't hear. Sometimes, the best way to understand the body is to **listen closely—literally from the inside.**

Mind-Blowing Medical Breakthrough #100

THE VACCINE THAT FIGHTS CANCER

In a groundbreaking clinical trial, scientists developed a **personalized mRNA cancer vaccine** that teaches the immune system to **target a patient's unique tumor mutations**—similar to how COVID-19 mRNA vaccines teach the body to fight viruses. By analyzing a patient's tumor, scientists create a custom-tailored vaccine that activates **T-cells to attack only cancer cells**. Early trials for melanoma and pancreatic cancer have shown **promising remission rates**, marking a bold new frontier: **vaccines not just to prevent illness, but to cure it.**

CONCLUSION

Congratulations! You've just explored *100 Mind-Blowing Medical Breakthroughs* — a journey through the jaw-dropping moments, surprising innovations, and life-changing discoveries that have reshaped what we thought was possible. From accidental cures to futuristic tech, these stories show that medicine is more than science — it's a constant quest to push the limits of what the human body and mind can overcome.

But here's the thing about medical breakthroughs — they never stop. For every fact you've just read, there are countless more being written in labs, hospitals, and unexpected corners of the world. Maybe this book sparked your curiosity about the future of healthcare, or maybe it simply gave you a deeper appreciation for how far we've come. Either way, the truth is clear: **the story of medicine is still being written — one breakthrough at a time**.

So as you close this book, don't think of it as the end. Think of it as a deep breath before the next discovery, a moment of awe before science takes another leap forward.

Until next time, stay curious, stay inspired, and remember: the most mind-blowing break-throughs might still be ahead.

ACKNOWLEDGEMENTS

Creating *100 Mind-Blowing Medical Break-throughs* has been a journey filled with awe, curiosity, and a deep appreciation for the people and ideas that continue to shape the future of medicine. While my name may be on the cover, this book wouldn't exist without the inspiration, support, and brilliance of so many others.

First, a heartfelt thank you to the scientists, doctors, nurses, inventors, and everyday heroes who've dedicated their lives to pushing the boundaries of what's possible. Your breakthroughs, whether born in a lab, an ER, or by total accident, have saved lives, changed lives, and sparked the stories that fill these pages.

To my family and friends—thank you for tolerating my excited rants about self-injecting pills, smart toilets, and robotic limbs. Your patience, encouragement, and enthusiastic "Wow, that's wild!" reactions kept this book (and me) moving forward.

To my readers—this book is for you. Whether you're a science lover, trivia junkie, or someone who just likes to say "Wait, what?!" out loud, thank you for taking this journey with me. Your curiosity is what keeps these stories alive and relevant.

And finally, to the world of medicine itself—thank you for being relentless, fascinating, and full of wonder. You've turned hope into healing and science into something nothing short of magical. I'm honored to share just a glimpse of your story.

Here's to breakthroughs, to the ones still to come, and to the incredible people who make the impossible... possible.

ABOUT THE AUTHOR

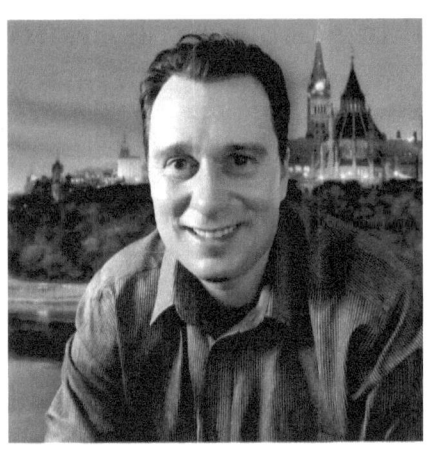

Felix Grayson is a storyteller at heart, driven by an insatiable curiosity for the strange, surprising, and downright unpredictable moments in science, medicine, and beyond. With a passion for uncovering the most astonishing and life-changing breakthroughs, Felix has crafted *100 Mind-Blowing Medical Breakthroughs* to entertain, inspire, and spark wonder in readers of all backgrounds.

When he's not diving deep into research or chasing down the next jaw-dropping discovery, Felix enjoys reading up on cutting-edge tech, wandering through science museums, and pondering life's most fascinating questions over a strong cup of coffee. A firm believer in the power of curiosity and the magic of a well-told fact, Felix invites you to explore the wild world of medical innovation—proof that truth really is stranger (and more amazing) than fiction.

www.ingramcontent.com/pod-product-compliance
Lightning Source LLC
Chambersburg PA
CBHW031310120626
46554CB00001BA/358